EAT GOOD TO FEEL GOOD

EAT GOOD TO FEEL GOOD

EAT GOOD TO FEEL GOOD

EAT GOOD TO FEEL GOOD

EAT GOOD TO FEEL GOOD

EAT GOOD TO FEEL GOOD

EAT GOOD TO FEEL GOOD

EAT GOOD TO FEEL GOOD

EAT GOOD TO FEEL GOOD

EAT GOOD TO FEEL GOOD

EAT GOOD TO FEEL GOOD

EAT GOOD TO FEEL GOOD

EAT GOOD TO FEEL GOOD

EAT GOOD TO FEEL GOOD

EAT GOOD TO FEEL GOOD

EAT GOOD TO FEEL GOOD

EAT GOOD TO FEEL GOOD

EAT GOOD TO FEEL GOOD

EAT GOOD TO FEEL GOOD
THE BATTLE BETWEEN GOOD AND EVIL....
ON OUR PLATE!

To contact the author/publisher, email
jenny@jbhealthcoach.com

ISBN-13: 978-1535004961
ISBN-10: 1535004967

Dedication

To the biggest super heroes in my life, my husband Jon, son Leo, and mom Susan.

Acknowledgement

**Thank you to my family and friends
for your support and encouragement!**

This Isn't Your Everyday Book!

Hey There! Before you start reading this book, I need to tell you a couple things.

This isn't the kind of book you just sit and read – you have to think, and answer questions.

There are no right or wrong answers though!

We are sharing information with each other.

There are times you will need to put the book down, and go do something before you can continue!

Maybe you've read a book like this.....or maybe you haven't. You won't know until you start, so let's go!

Super Heroes and **Villains**, Yeah, You Know Them!

Let me guess, you've heard about all kinds of Super Heroes (good guys) and Villains (bad guys), right? I bet you know more than me!

First question for you, **what makes a Super Hero a good guy?** Take your time to answer before reading on.

Okay, my turn. I think that Super Heroes save people from danger and help when people are hurt or sick. Did we have the same ideas?

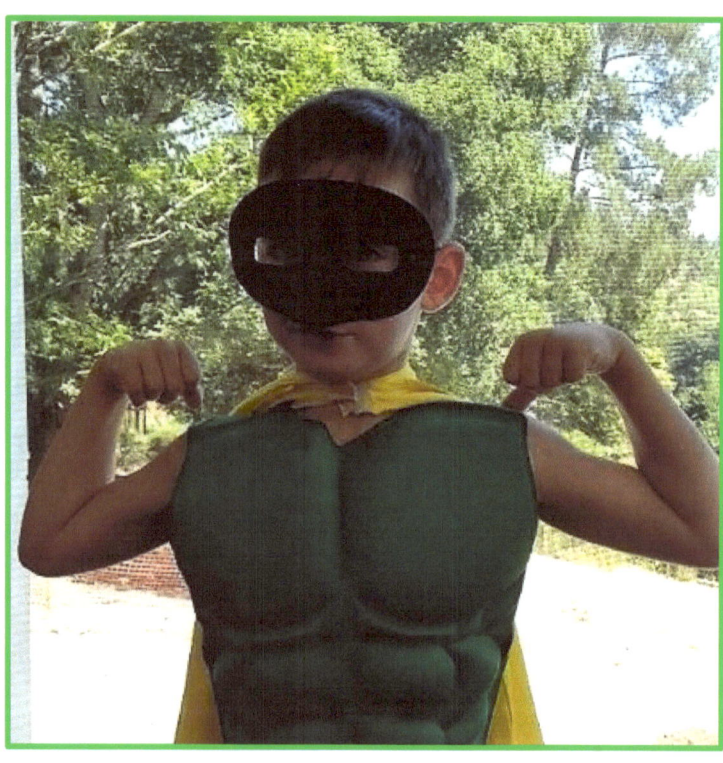

Next question, **what makes Villains bad guys?**

Let's compare ideas again! I think that Villains put people in danger and hurt them, and lie and trick people to get what they want.

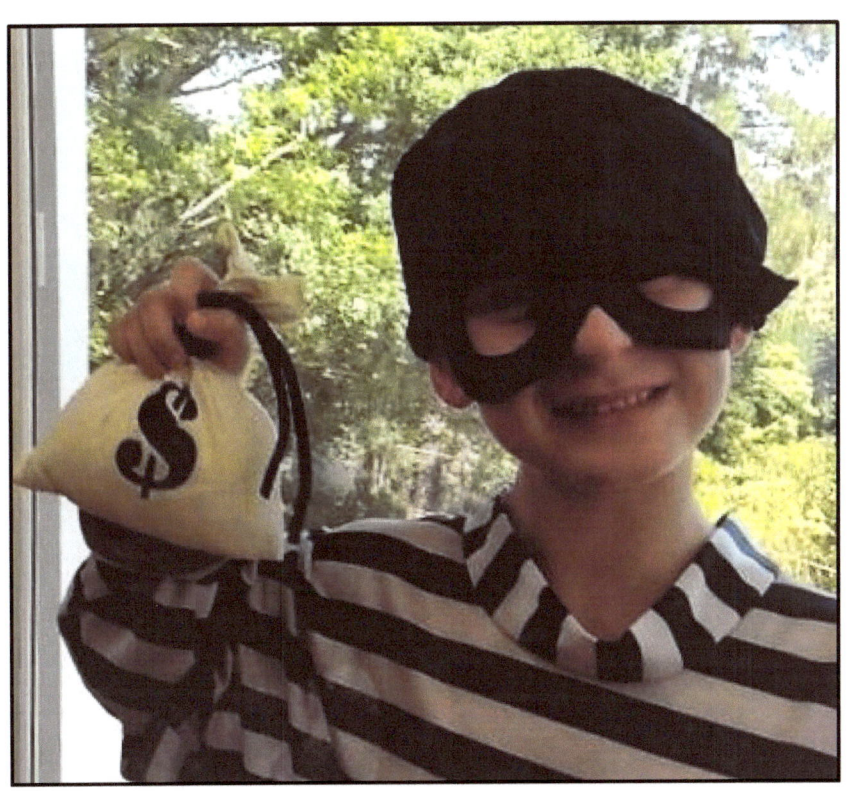

And, **what do Villains usually want?**

LOTS and LOTS of MONEY (**$$$$$**), which gives them LOTS and LOTS of POWER!

How did I do?

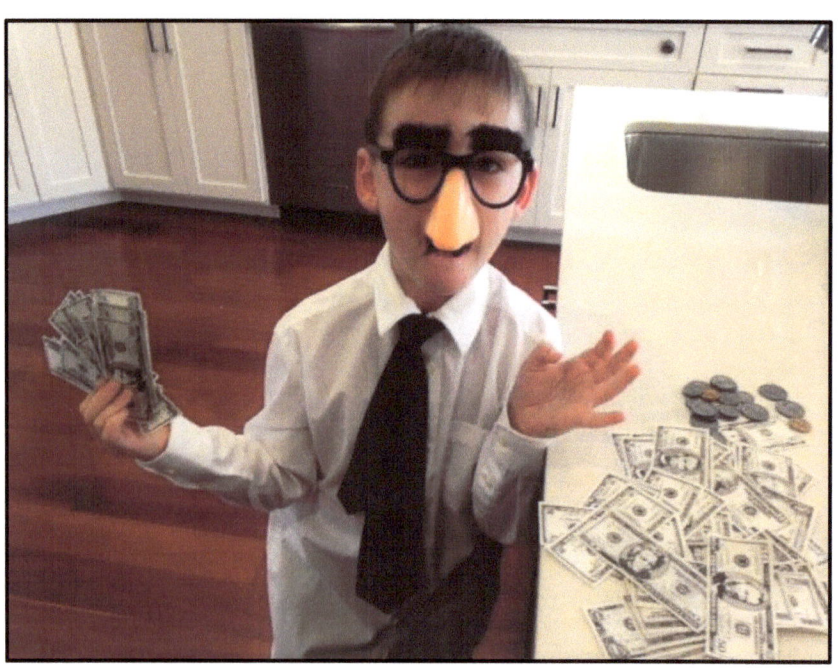

Good Vs Evil....In Our Body!

This might seem like a crazy question, but **do you think there are Super Heroes and Villains in the food we eat?**

I hope you said yes, because **there sure are** Super Heroes and Villains in the food we eat!

So, what makes food a Super Hero?

Let's compare our ideas! Here's what I think about Super Hero Food:

- ➤ Gives us energy
- ➤ Helps us grow
- ➤ Makes us smarter
- ➤ Keeps us from getting sick
- ➤ Makes our tummies feel good
- ➤ Helps our eyes see better and our skin feel softer
- ➤ Makes our nails and hair grow
- ➤ Makes our teeth and bones strong
- ➤ Makes us feel happy!

Now, what makes food a **Villain?**

Time to compare again! I think Villain food:

> ➢ Makes us get tired quickly when playing outside, running around, playing sports, and trying to concentrate at school
> ➢ Gives us tummy aches
> ➢ **Tricks our bodies into wanting to eat more and more and MORE, so we eat too much and don't feel good**
> ➢ **Makes our skin bumpy and itchy and gives us cavities in our teeth**
> ➢ Tricks us again by tasting REALLY good, but making our bodies and minds WEAK
> ➢ **Makes us get very sick and need to go to the doctor for medicine**

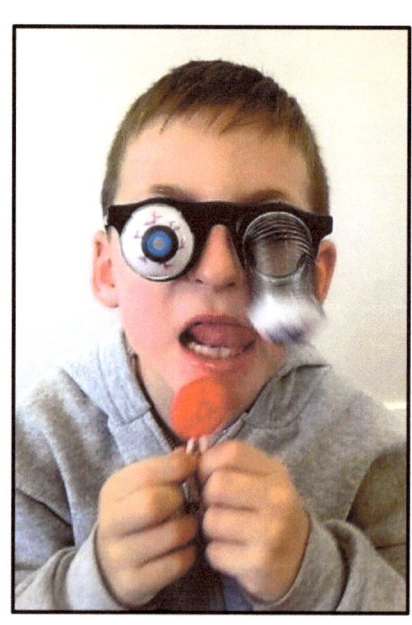

Here's another question for you, **if Villain food hurts us so much, why can we buy it?** This is a tough question, so think about it before answering!

Here's what I think - Villain food is like all the other Villains we talked about:

Villain food makes money for the people who sell it, and Villains want LOTS of money (**$$$$$**) to have LOTS of power. It gets even worse! Villain food might sometimes cost less to buy than Super Hero food, but eventually, it costs a lot more money for the people that eat it.

How is that possible? Here's the sneaky part, after eating too much Villain food, people have to spend more money to go to doctors when they get sick, to dentists when they get cavities, and to buy lots of medicine to make their bodies feel better.

Talk about evil!

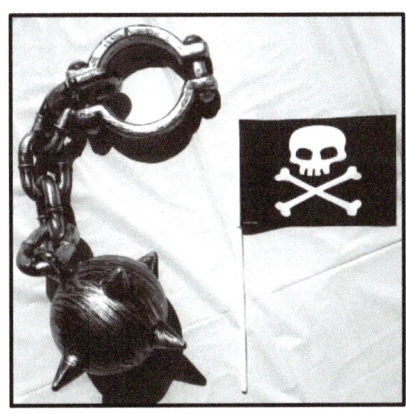

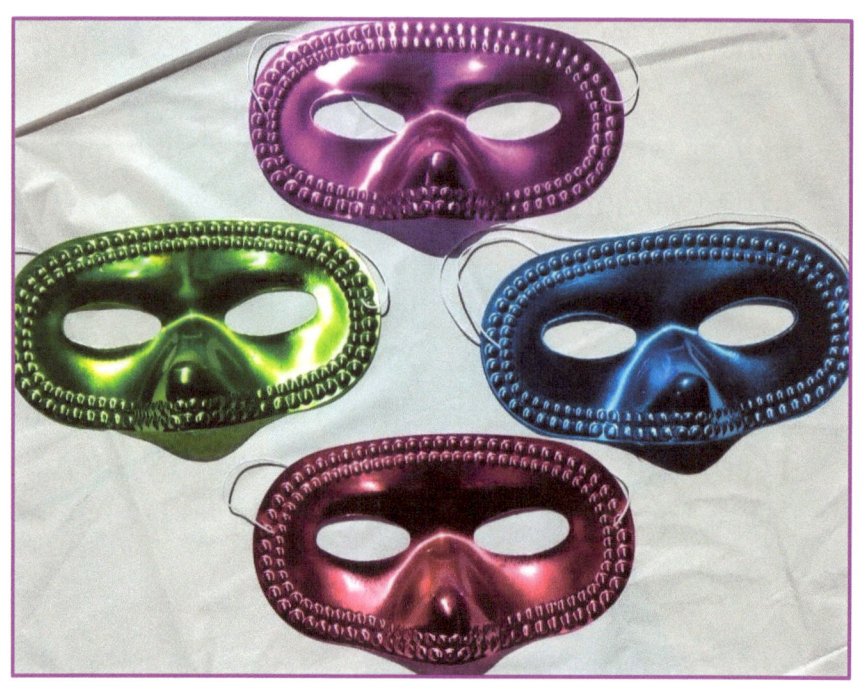

The Masks Come Off!

What kind of food are we talking about?

The best Super Hero food comes from nature!

Some categories of Super Hero food include fruit, vegetables, beans, whole grains, like brown rice, farro, and quinoa (keen-wah), and food that comes from animals, like milk, cheese, eggs, chicken, beef, turkey, and fish.

Are you wondering if it's okay to eat food from animals? That's a great question! Some people choose to only eat food that comes from plants. Many people feel very good when they eat food from animals, so it's okay for them.

If you choose to eat food from animals, it is very important to make sure the animals were given lots of good care, freedom to move around outside, and fed the right healthy food for them. When an animal is treated well, healthy, and lives a happy life, the food that comes from it and goes in your body is better for you!

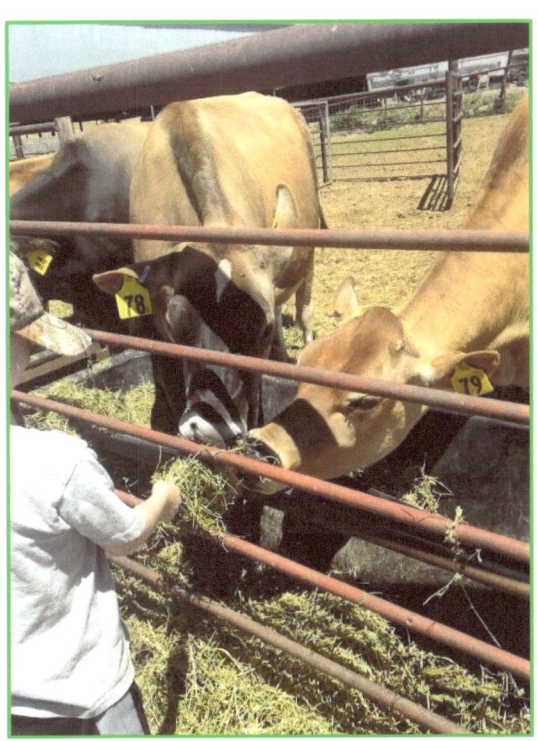

What else makes food a Super Hero?

Food that has lots of vitamins and minerals that keep our bodies, hearts, and brains healthy. Also, food that is high in fiber helps our tummies feel good!

What about Villain food?

Villain food is not grown in nature, and is usually in packaged boxes, bags, jars, and bottles, with a LONG list of ingredients that have LOTS of letters and are very hard to read and say out loud. Villain food usually has a lot of added sugar in it to disguise the taste of yucky things that are put in the food to make it look better and last a very LONG time.

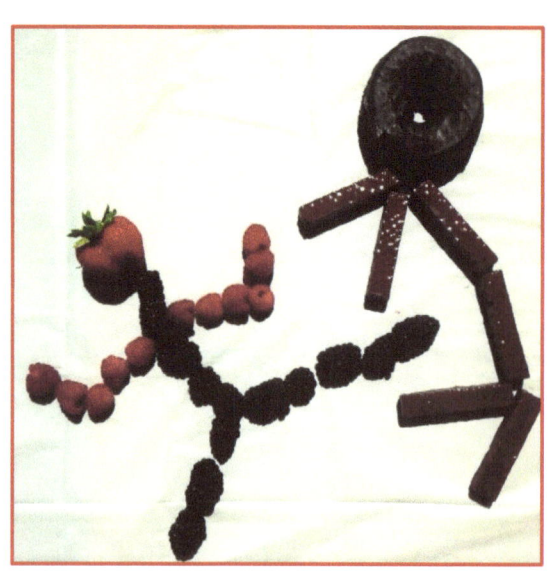

Your First Mission!

Now it's time for something really different! I'm going to give you an assignment, actually a special mission. You need to know some information first:

A fast way to decide whether packaged food (in a box, bag, jar, etc.) is a Super Hero or a Villain is to look at the words **Sugar** and **Fiber** on the label and see what number is next to the word. For your mission, food that is **HIGH in FIBER** and **LOW in SUGAR** will be a **Super Hero food** and food that is **LOW in FIBER** and **HIGH in SUGAR** will be a Villain food.

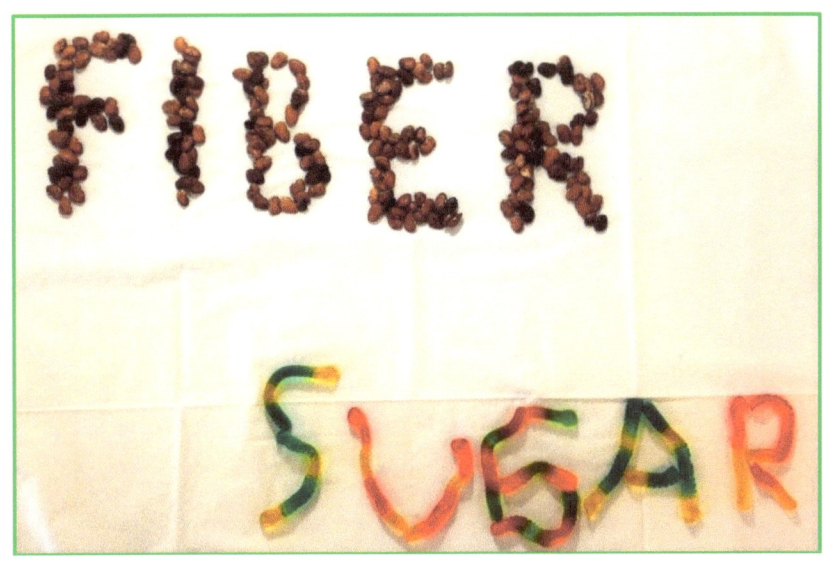

Here are your instructions – follow them carefully:

Go in your kitchen and examine the food labels and decide what is a **Super Hero food** and what is a **Villain food**.

Pay careful attention to the designs on the boxes, bags, etc. Think about if there are certain designs (like super heroes, movie, and TV characters) that make you want to buy and eat that food?

Look at what foods come from nature, like fruit, vegetables, whole grains, eggs, milk, and the other categories we talked about earlier.

Once you are finished, come back and let's discuss what you found!

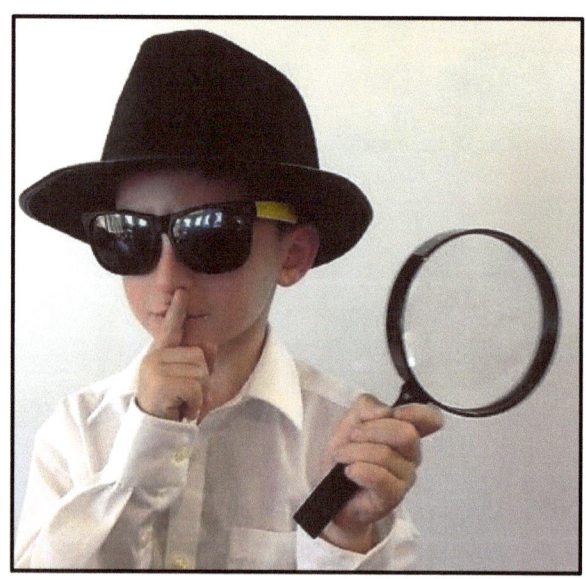

What Did You Find?

Is your mission complete? I'm so excited to hear about what you found!

What food did you find that came from nature and what were your favorites? Was there any **Super Hero food** from nature you wish you had? If yes, <u>add it to the next shopping list!</u>

What **Super Hero food** did you find that were in boxes, bags, jars, etc. that were **LOW in SUGAR** and **HIGH in FIBER**, and what were your favorites?

What **Villain food** did you find that were **HIGH in SUGAR** and **LOW in FIBER**? What were your favorites…..and don't try and tell me you don't have a favorite villain food. We all do, so let's be honest. **Nobody is perfect!**

What food had the **most sugar**?

What food had the **most fiber**?

Tell me about the packages!

Were there packages that had Super Heroes on them or other characters from TV or movies?

Were they **Super Hero** or **Villain food**?

Do you think that Villain food tries to look fun for kids so you want to buy it when you are shopping? **Could that be another sneaky villain trick?** I think so!

Do you think you need **more Super Hero food? Why or why not?**

Do you think you have **too much Villain food? Why or why not?**

Your Next Mission!

I hope you don't think you're done, because you have a new mission! You don't have to go anywhere for this one though.

Here is a very important question:

Could you stop buying and eating any of the **Villain food** you found, and replace it with a **Super Hero food** that tastes just as good, and is much better for you?

Pick **at least one** swap for your mission, and **try it out for 3 weeks. Mark the days on your calendar, then tell me how you did!**

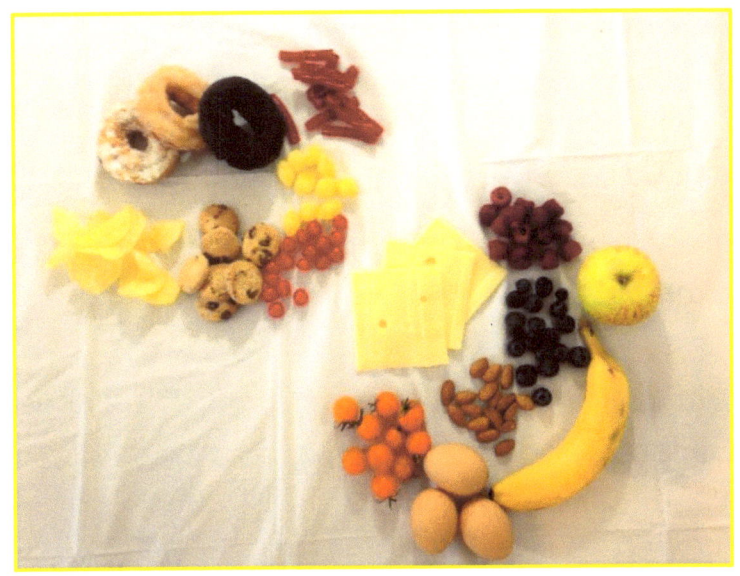

Create Your Own Teams of Super Hero and Villain Food, and Go To Battle!

Now it's time for you to get really creative! We discussed some of your favorite Super Hero and Villain food, and you know about Super Heroes and Villains in stories, TV shows, and movies, but.....have you ever created your own?

Your next mission, the most important yet, is first to create a team of Super Hero food and give them names! **Pick at least three** Super Hero foods that you love, and then have fun giving them names! Here's a few ideas I had:

Super Spinach * Captain Kale *
Awesome Avocado
Fantastic Farro * **Brawny Black Beans**
Stunning Strawberries * Wonder Water

Next, what Villain food will you have a hard time giving up? Give them names! Here are a few examples:

Sneaky Sugar * Cunning Candy * Devious Donuts
Sinister Soda * Menacing Marshmallows
Cruel Caramel

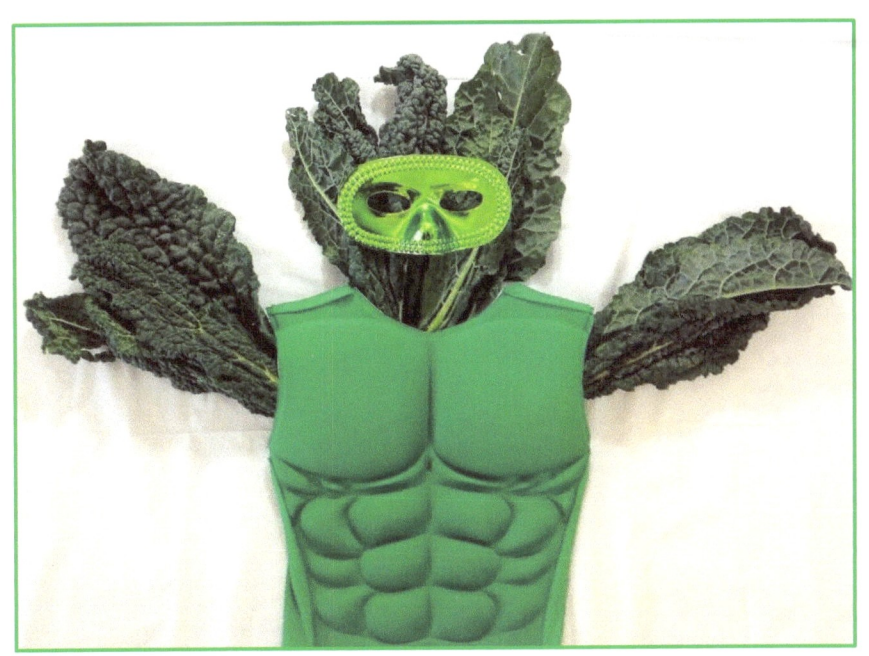

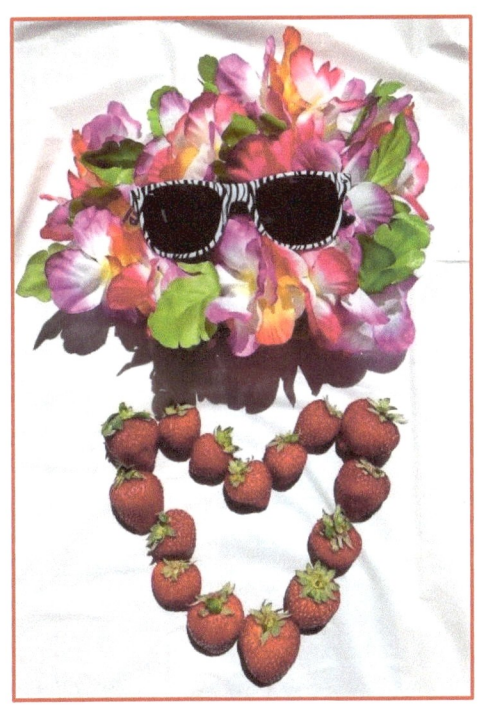

Now that you assembled your Super Hero food team, they can battle the Villain food when you are tempted to the dark side of the plate!

You are what you eat, so
eat good to feel good!

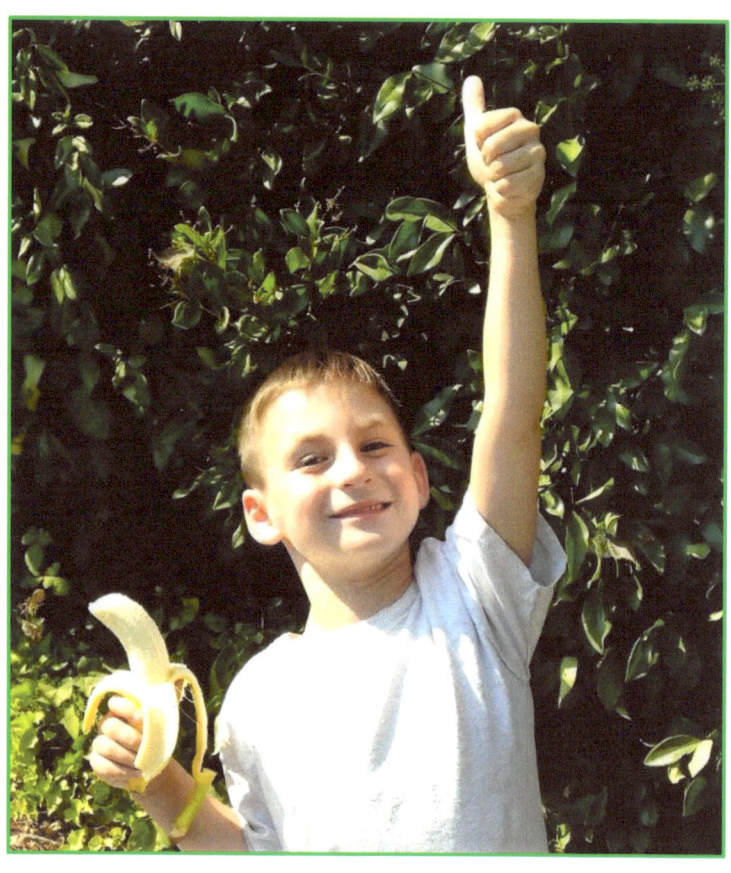

About the Author

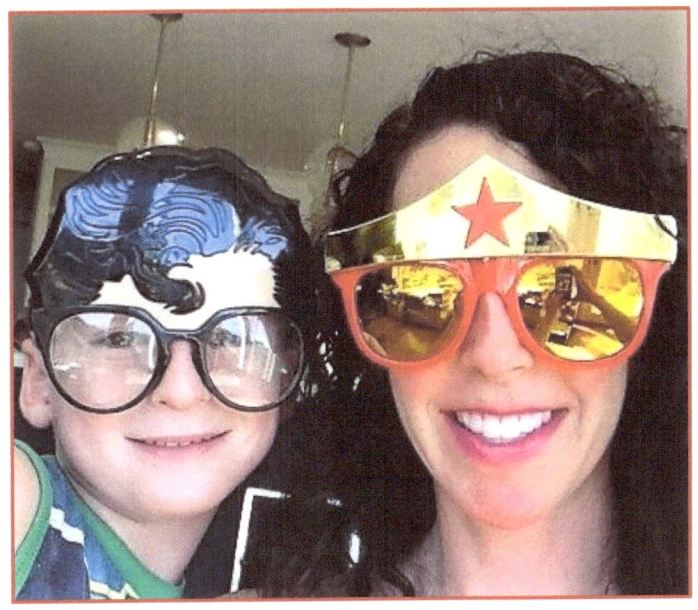

Jenny Bergschneider is a health coach with a passion for helping families and children. She lives in Northern California with her husband and son. If she had to name one of each, her favorite super hero food would be avocados and her favorite villain food would be ice cream. For an easy super hero food meal that also satisfies a sweet tooth, she loves a baked sweet potato topped with cottage cheese and cinnamon – YUM!

EAT GOOD TO FEEL GOOD

EAT GOOD TO FEEL GOOD

EAT GOOD TO FEEL GOOD

EAT GOOD TO FEEL GOOD

EAT GOOD TO FEEL GOOD

EAT GOOD TO FEEL GOOD

EAT GOOD TO FEEL GOOD

EAT GOOD TO FEEL GOOD

EAT GOOD TO FEEL GOOD

EAT GOOD TO FEEL GOOD

EAT GOOD TO FEEL GOOD

EAT GOOD TO FEEL GOOD

EAT GOOD TO FEEL GOOD

EAT GOOD TO FEEL GOOD

EAT GOOD TO FEEL GOOD

EAT GOOD TO FEEL GOOD

EAT GOOD TO FEEL GOOD

EAT GOOD TO FEEL GOOD

www.ingramcontent.com/pod-product-compliance
Lightning Source LLC
Chambersburg PA
CBHW050931290526
45792CB00002B/968